FIRST AID ON THE FARM

Natural and Conventional Treatments

By
Alfred L. Anduze
And
Ferdinand Rivera Villalba

iUniverse books may be ordered through booksellers or by contacting:

iUniverse
1663 Liberty Drive
Bloomington, IN 47403
www.iuniverse.com
1-800-Authors (1-800-288-4677)

Because of the dynamic nature of the Internet, any web addresses or links contained in this book may have changed since publication and may no longer be valid. The views expressed in this work are solely those of the author and do not necessarily reflect the views of the publisher, and the publisher hereby disclaims any responsibility for them.

Any people depicted in stock imagery provided by Thinkstock are models, and such images are being used for illustrative purposes only.
Certain stock imagery © Thinkstock.

ISBN: 978-1-5320-1947-0 (sc)
ISBN: 978-1-5320-1948-7 (e)

Library of Congress Control Number: 2017905030

Print information available on the last page.

iUniverse rev. date: 04/26/2017

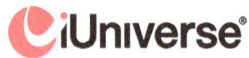

Acknowledgements (first aid emergency guides)
(Saluan Farm workbook of natural health)
Illustrations by Jaye Thompson

Emergency phone numbers...

Ambulance...   911_____

Doctor........._____

Poison control...1 800 222 1222

Hospital... _____

Police ..._____

Fire ..._____

Electric or gas co..._____

Suicide hotline ... 1 800 273 8255

Domestic abuse.... 1 800 799 7233

Contents

Introduction

First aid is the emergency medical care given before professional care is available. In most cases it is sufficient for complete recovery. In some cases it is essential for stabilization while complete medical care is on the way. Why the farm? It is often located in a remote area, away from adequate medical facilities, with high exposure to sun, insects, reptiles, poisonous plants, wind, dust, and variable temperatures. Farming activities are highly susceptible to accidents due to use of tools, machinery, animal care, difficult terrain and use of cleaning materials which may lead to a higher incidence of infections from bacteria, viruses, fungi and parasites.

The purpose of this book is to provide a quick easy guide to the recognition and treatment of basic emergency conditions that may be encountered on a farm in the tropics.

*In addition to the conventional treatments and medications, this book contains natural treatments using products that may be present on the farm and surrounding forests.

Dr Ferdinand Rivera Villalba is a practicing podiatrist in Mayaguez and experienced farmer in Maricao, Puerto Rico.

Dr Alfred Lee Anduze is a retired ophthalmologist, medicinal plant specialist, and farmer in Maricao, Puerto Rico.

Mr. Jaye Thompson is a student of graphic design at the University of Delaware, USA.

Basic First Aid kit

A. Supplies:

Sterile adhesive bandages (various sizes),
Non-stick gauze bandages
Adhesive cloth tape,
Absorbent compress dressing
Antiseptic wipes
Band-Aids,
Bandage roll
Cold pack (instant),
Heat pad
Gauze pads (sterile)
Butterfly closures
Scissors,
Oral thermometer
Triangular arm sling
Tweezers (plastic)
Cotton tip applicators (sterile)
Eye pads
Blanket
Crutches

B. Cleansers:

Antibacterial liquid soap in dispenser
Antiseptic solution & wipes,
Alcohol pads,
Hydrogen peroxide 3%
Witch hazel

Sterile eyewash
Gloves (non-latex)

C. Medications: External

Antibiotic ointment (bacitracin, polysporin, neomycin)
Antibiotic herbals (*calendula oil, papaya latex, tarragon, thyme, verveine)

Aloe Vera cream	(burn and sting treatment)
Arnica or curia	(bruise, contusion treatment)
Hydrocortisone 2.5% ointment,	(inflammation control & itch relief)
Silvadene 1% cream	(burn treatment)
Lemongrass, Geraniol or Neem oil	(insect repellant)
Eucalyptus or pennyroyal oil	(insect bite treatment)
Tincture of yarrow	(bleeding control)
Tea tree oil, miconazole or clotrimazole	(fungal treatment)
Lidocaine/ethyl alcohol, stinging nettle oil	(sting & allergy rash relief)
Cortaid, calamine lotion, noni oil	(itch relief),
Mentholated muscle cream or rub, arnica	(muscle strain, sprain, soreness relief)
Cloves	(toothache and antibiotic)
Diphenhydramine cream	(antihistamine allergy rash relief)
Baking soda (sodium bicarbonate)	(insect bite treatment)

oils for topical use can be made by boiling and mixing natural ingredients with olive, grape seed, or canola oil base

Internal:

Epinephrine single dose, 1:1000,(0.3%) 1 cc.	(Pre-loaded syringe) Epi-pen
Sublingual epinephrine tablets 40 mg.	(Severe allergic reaction)
Aspirin, acetoaminophen	(acute fever and pain relief)
Turmeric	(chronic inflammation and painkiller)
Ipecac syrup	(acute poisoning, induce vomiting)
Antacid, Ginger, chamomile	(indigeston, nausea relief)

Diphenhydramine capsules 25 mg   (allergic reaction)
Antiviral herbals   (artemesia, basil, anamú, chamomile, lemongrass, peppermint)

Basic Accident Prevention:

Be aware of unsafe acts and conditions when operating equipment and using tools; wear safety attire when indicated; follow instructions; stay dry and dress appropriately for all activities; be aware of acts of nature and take necessary precautions.

Condition/...What to do in case of this situation?

There are three categories of injury or illness. Mild afflictions are self- limited and will usually heal with minimum care and time. Moderate conditions can be treated in place. Some may need further medical attention and will be designated as *seek medical care. Severe situations are life threatening and will be designated as **seek medical help, medical facility required.

Assess the problem and start the treatment.

A.Mild:
(temporarily incapacitating; self-limited)

1. Too Hot : Dehydration:

a. Heat exhaustion: old, wet, clammy skin, fatigue

Put person in cool, shaded place, elevate feet, apply cool wet cloths to skin, drink cool water

b. Heat stroke: hot, flushed, dry skin, with or without fever

(Put person to *lie down in cool shaded area, apply cold water or ice pack to to neck.*)

seek medical care immediately

2. Too Cold:

a. hypothermia: low body temperature, shivering, drowsy, numb

Move person to a warm area, dress warm dry clothing, wrap in blanket or towels, may

coddle the person in order to add own body heat, use a fire or vehicle engine heat, drink warm non-alcoholic drinks with electrolytes,

*seek medical care immediately

B. frostbite: area turns white and numb,

Warm affected area with clothing or warm water, cover with warm sterile dressings,

*seek medical care immediately

3. Digestion problems

a. Stomachache/indigestion: (*natural tea of ginger, chamomile, spearmint, peppermint, cayenne, goatweed and sage, or any combination of these herbals.*)

b. Constipation: (*cascara sagrada, Metamucil, psyllium, Aloe Vera, cinnamon*)

c. Diarrhea: (*black tea, tea of curia (Tilo)*)

4. Infections:

A. Bacterial: a farm environment may lead to increased exposure and susceptibility to infectious organisms. Example: Leptospirosis is a bacterial disease contracted through contact with food, water or soil contaminated with infected animal urine. Persistent symptoms of high fever, chills, headache, red eyes, stomach pain, diarrhea and/or vomiting of more than 3 days, should *seek medical help

> B.   Viral: Colds and flu are mainly due to viruses and are self-limited: *(symptoms are best treated with increased intake of water/fluids/and natural tea:*
>
> *Mix spearmint, ginger, rosemary, dandelion, anamú, artemesia, garlic, basil, and/or lemongrass)*

C.   *Fungal: Many invasive organisms reside in warm, moist humid areas like old dead decaying plant and tree matter. Infections of the feet, crotch, armpits, hair and ears are common and can be avoided by washing these areas well with soap and warm water and drying well. Mild to moderate involvements respond to tea tree oil, miconazole and/or clotrimazole applications.*

5. Skin rash:

allergic reaction to (plants, pollen, grass, molds, chemicals, smoke, food (tree nuts, peanuts, mangoes, tomatoes, milk, soy, wheat, eggs, shellfish, animal dander): sudden appearance of redness, warm skin, itching, formation of bumps and wheals (external.)

Treat acute allergy (mild) : cold compress, apply hydrocortisone ointment and/or stinging nettle oil,

If moderate, take oral Benadryl 25 mg and one cup of chamomile tea

If severe (extensive swelling, difficult breathing, weakness), put the victim to lie down, face up, open the airway, check vital signs, give a sublingual epinephrine tablet (under tongue), or Epi-pen injection.(see anaphylaxis)

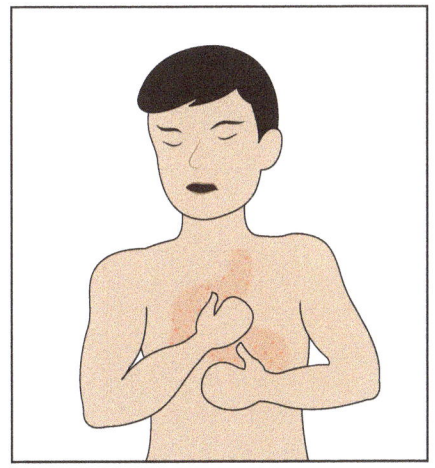

Skin rash

6. Superficial trauma:

cuts & scrapes ...infection is high risk in a tropical setting due to dampness, humidity, heat/cold drafts : no injury is insignificant (*wash with soap and water, apply hydrogen peroxide, antibiotic ointment, aloe vera gel, band-aid optional; mild to moderate infections may respond to natural applications of cinnamon, papaya latex, and calendula, noni, neem oils.*)

B. Moderate: (limb or organ threatening; infection possible)

General wound care (antisepsis...disinfection...sterilization)
Clean, cover, protect, prevent infection, promote healing

1. Abscess_ do not cover; *clean with alcohol wipes, apply warm compress,*
seek medical care for drainage if no improvement in 24 hours

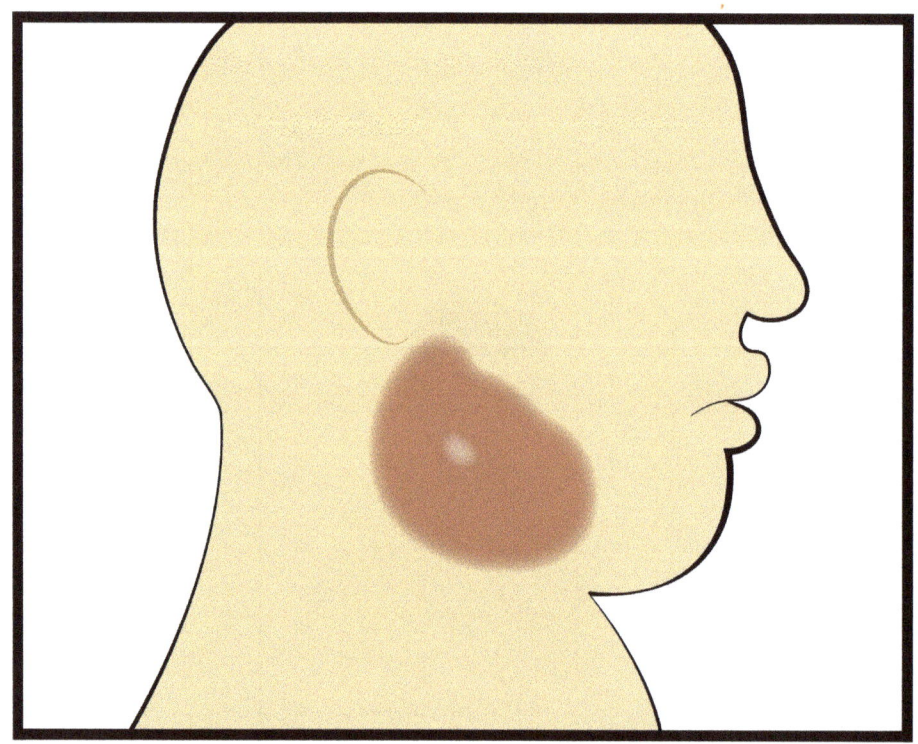

7. Abrasion:
skin scraped off, large area red

Wash with soap & water, apply peroxide and antibiotic ointment or calendula oil, apply sterile gauze, inspect and change gauze often.

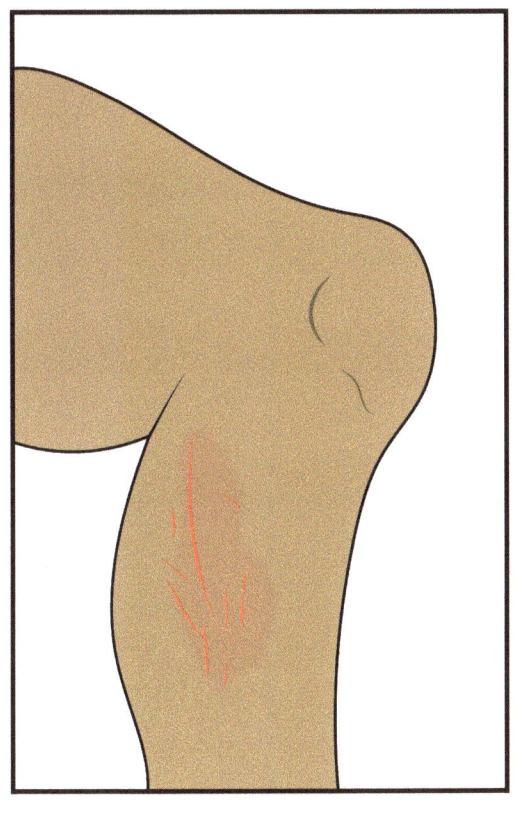

Scrapes

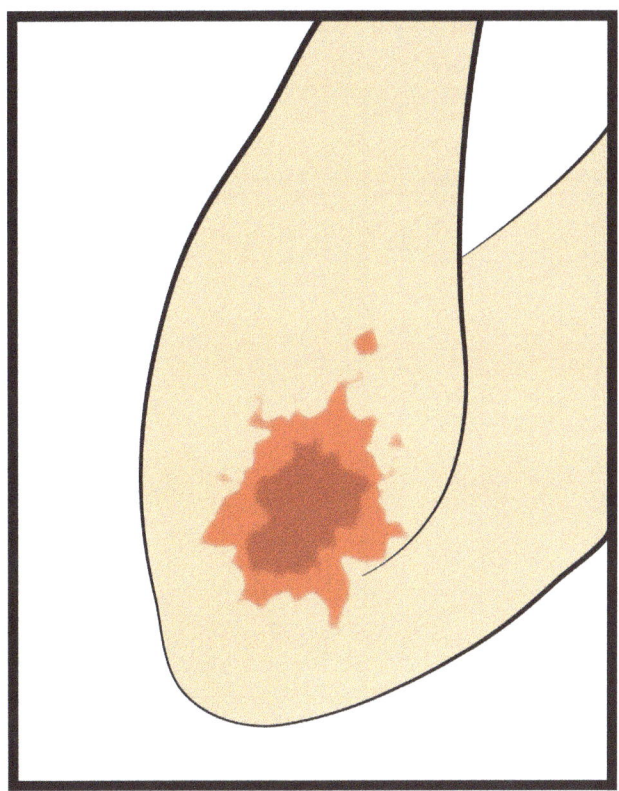

Elbow skin scraped off

8.Bruises:

skin intact, soft tissue damage; contusion; discolored skin (blood capillaries ruptured), *apply cold pack several times a day (not directly to skin)for 1-2 days to constrict blood vessels and reduce swelling,then apply hot pack or warm moist cloth to promote blood flow and healing. Witch hazel solution, arnica or curia may also be applied.*

*Seek medical help if no improvement after 3 days. Avoid aspirin ibuprofen and other blood thinners.

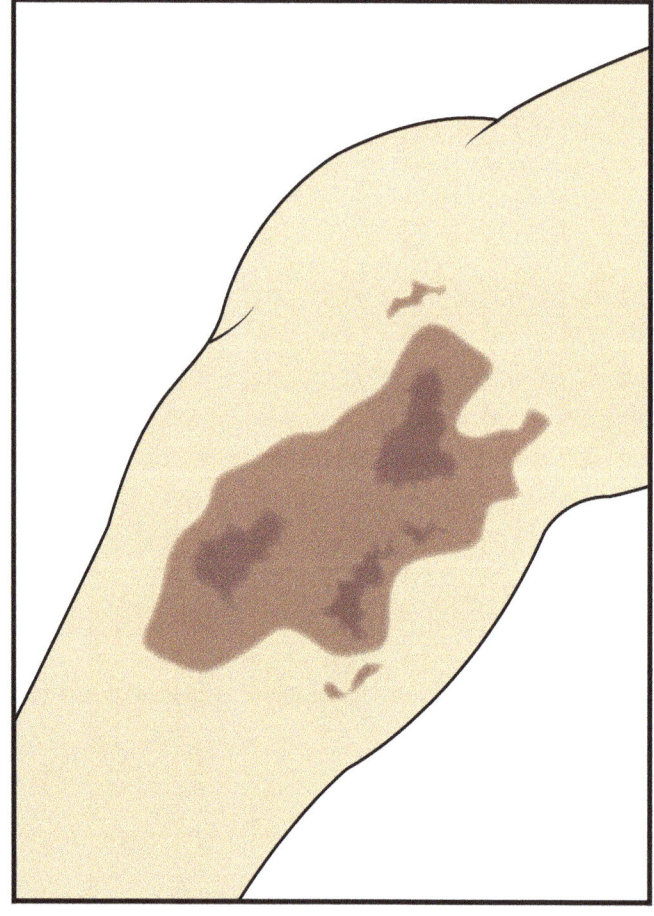

Bruise on the leg calf

9. Bites and stings:

A.   Mosquitos, sanguinos, flies, fleas, ticks, no-see-ums, ants…

Bite Prevention: 1. remain indoors at dusk
2. Loose fitting clothing, long sleeves, tuck pants into socks,
3. Avoid black or white fabrics (attraction)
4. Outdoor fan or breezy area
5. Natural insect repellent with geraniol, neem oil, lemongrass, lemonbalm, cinnamon, catnip,

Treatment: After bite: *apply aloe vera oil with Vitamin E, tea tree oil, basil, lemongrass, peppermint, noni, eucalyptus, pennyroyal, soybean oils for skin*

B. Bee, wasp and centipede: immediate pain and swelling.

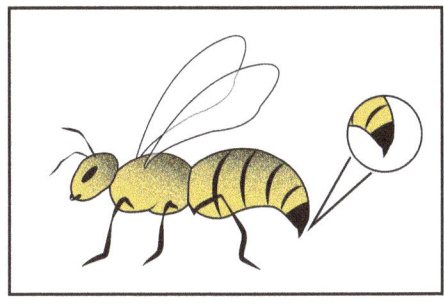 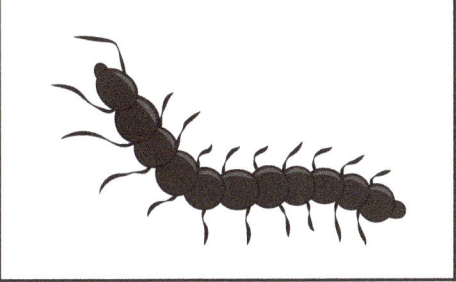 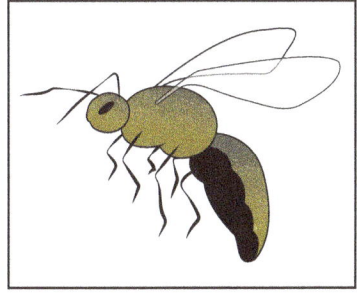

Bee   Wasp   Centipede

Try to remove stinger by scraping it off, do not squeeze or may release more venom, wash area with soap and water, apply cold compress (not ice) to reduce swelling, apply cortaid, hydrocortisone cream or calamine lotion for itch and pain, if severe, immerse area in cold water with baking soda / take benadryl capsule if moderate to severe. Do not rub or scratch will worsen itching and pain...

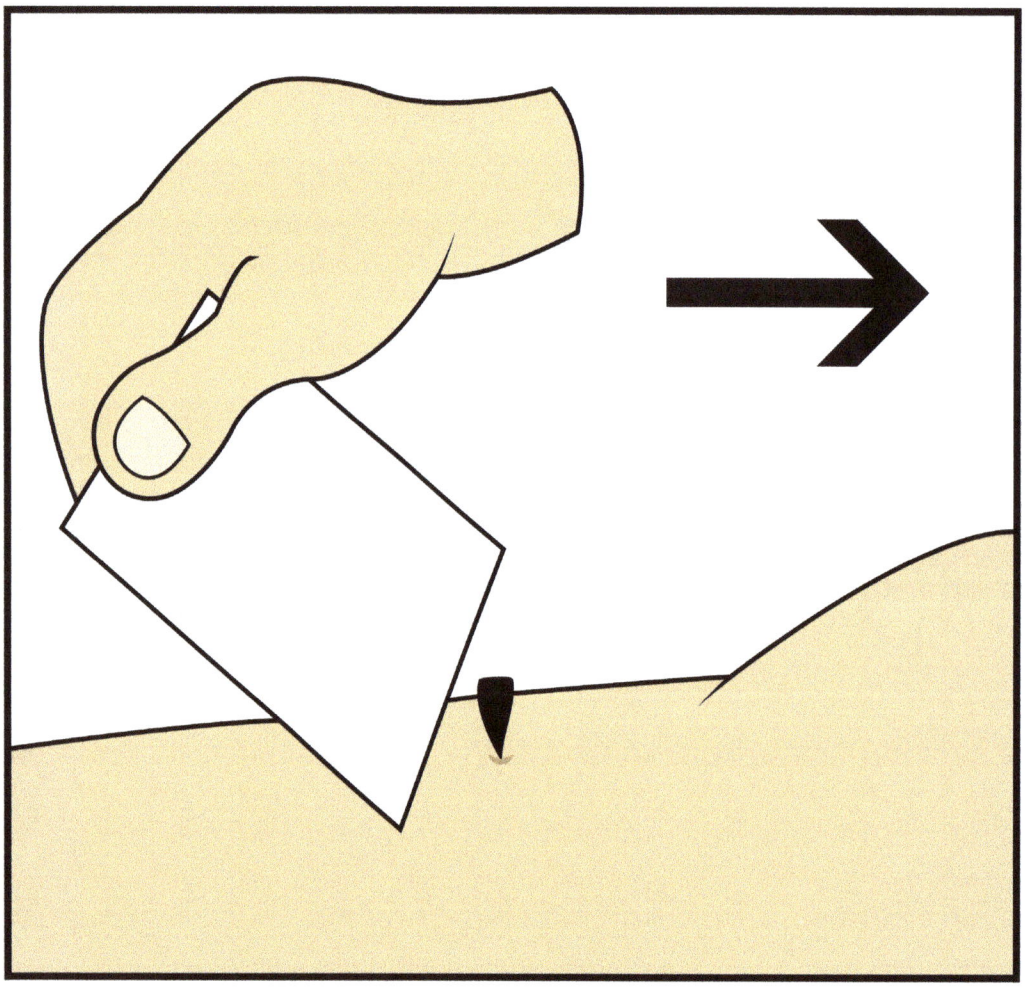

Remove stinger with a card

E. Spider: there is no initial pain, redness and itch develop gradually. *Early: treat itch with cortaid or calamine lotion, & cold pack to slow spread of poison. Late if painful ulcer appears, use warm compress and antibiotic cream.*

Watch for anaphylaxis reaction.

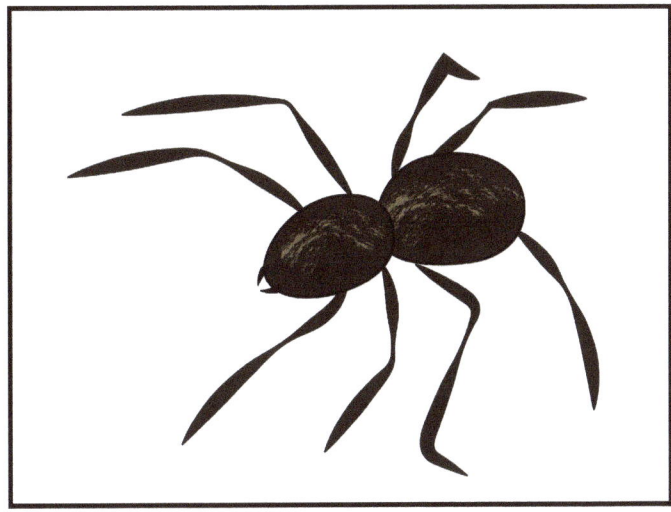

Spider

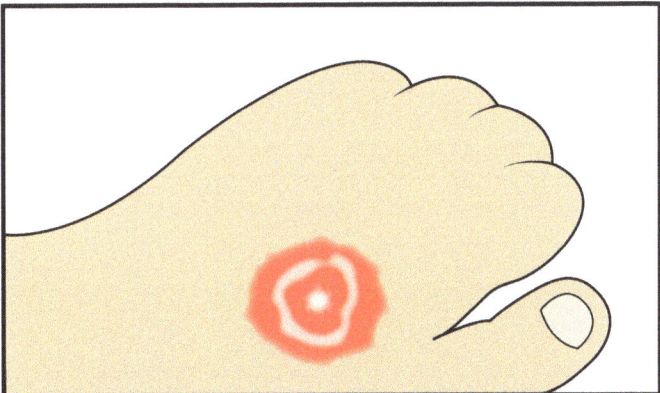

Spider bite pustule ulcer on foot

Anaphylaxis: *severe reaction to stings, bites, poisons, drugs, food or chemical toxins... sudden onset of swelling, redness, rash (hives), weakness, nausea, vomiting, dizziness, breathing difficulty, coughing, wheezing... _administer_ Epi-pen injection to thigh or upper arm or give epinephrine tablet under the tongue (faster absorption). *call for medical help immediately, wrap in blanket to induce sweating that may eliminate toxin through the pores.*

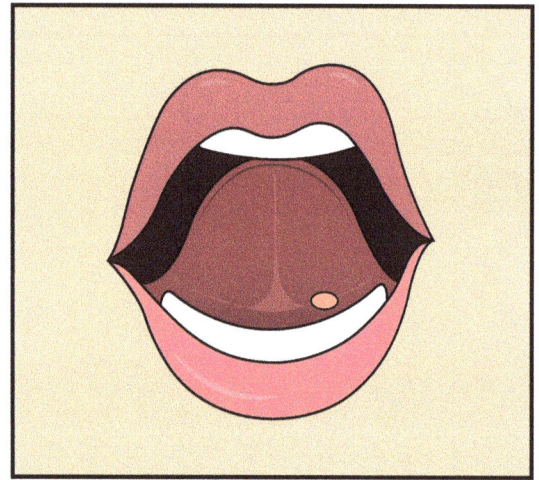

Sublingual tablet (open mouth, red lips)

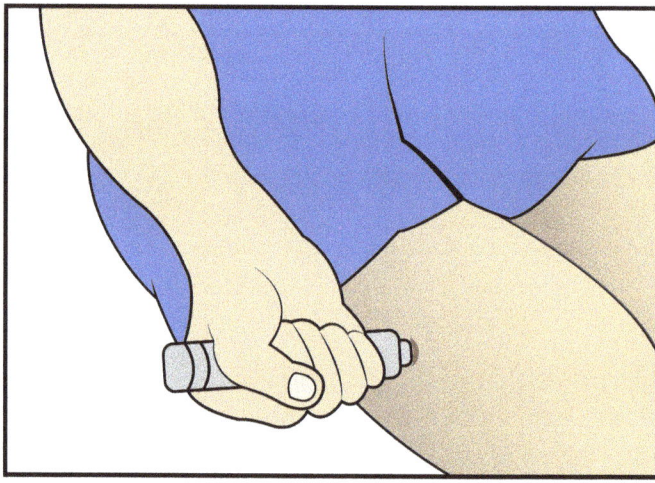

Epi-pen to the thigh

10. Impaled objects

A. **Splinter**: if small with protruding end, (*use tweezers to remove and apply hydrogen peroxide*) if deep (*apply peroxide, remove with heated needle and reapply peroxide and antibiotic ointment after removal) if difficult, *seek medical care*)

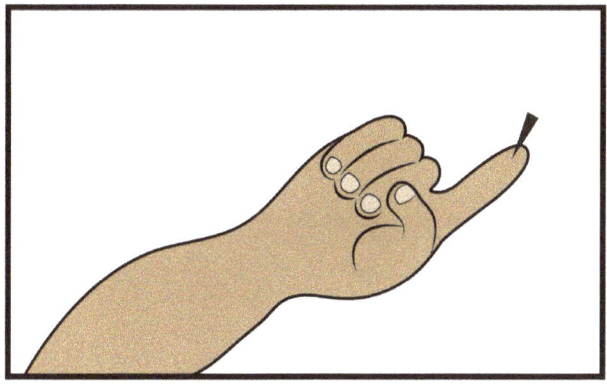

Splinter in finger

B. **Large object**/ penetration and protrusion: *do not remove; control bleeding, stabilize with thick dressing, *seek medical care.*

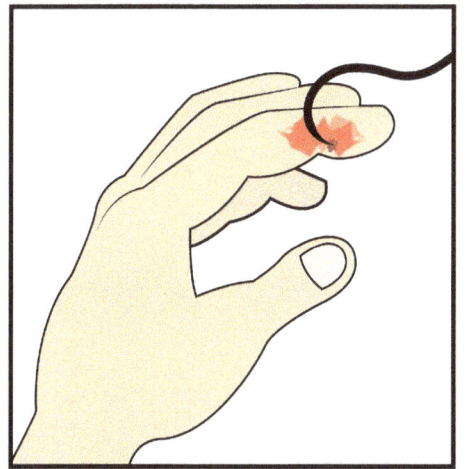

Hook in finger

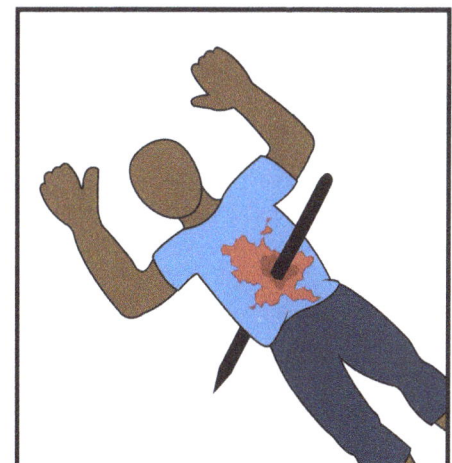

Impaled stake through the body

11. Open wound:

apply pressure to control bleeding, elevate above the level of the heart

A.Laceration:

cut, broken skin, loss of skin

(Cleanse with soap & water, alcohol pads, antiseptic wipes, control bleeding, apply direct pressure on wound with clean cloth or gauze, apply tincture of yarrow soaked gauze for clotting, do not remove soaked gauze, add new gauze and apply more pressure until bleeding stops...then apply sterile dressing.

(Small, closed wound) Apply peroxide for antisepsis, disinfection, sterilization warm pack or compress, antibiotic ointment or calendula oil, cover with bandage,

(Large, open wound) Elevate the limb or body part & apply cold compress to reduce pain & swelling, pressure for bleeding, lay strips of fresh papaya peel with latex onto the wound, butterfly closure if gaping, apply pressure bandage if bleeding continues, if bleeding persists or if wound remains open,

*seek medical care.

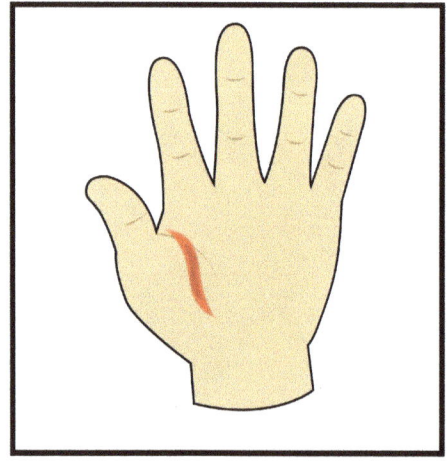

Hand laceration

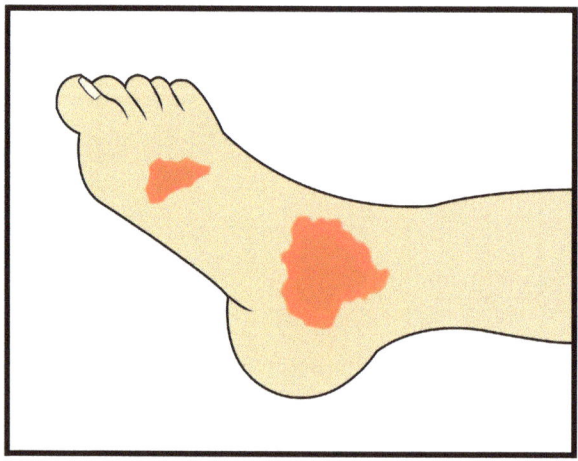

avulsions on the foot

B. Burns

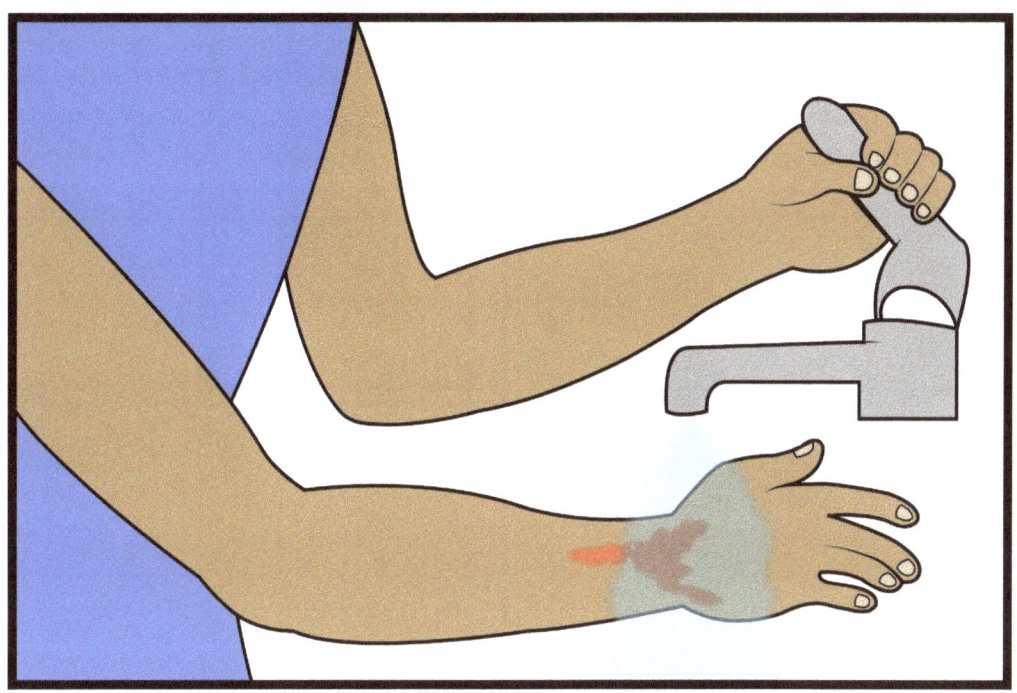

1st degree: superficial skin, mild pain, redness
(Wash gently, apply aloe vera cream or oil, acetaminophen for pain)

2nd degree: red, swollen/wet skin, considerable pain
(rinse in cool water X 15-30 minutes, apply cool compress (not ice), do not break blisters, cleanse with mild soap & water, pat dry with sterile gauze, apply antibiotic or silvadene cream or calendula oil (do not use butter or sprays as they trap heat), apply loose bandage if skin is broken, no tape. If the bandage sticks to skin, apply warm water to release it, do not encircle a limb (it needs good circulation)

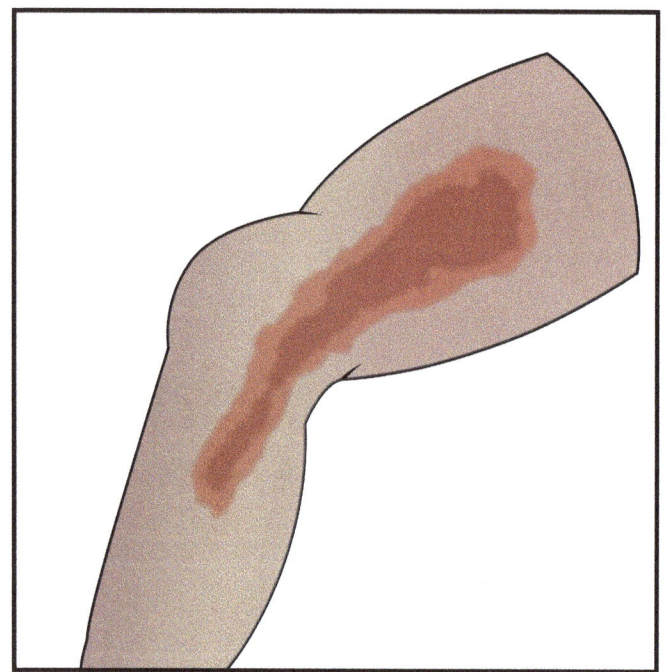

Second degree leg burn

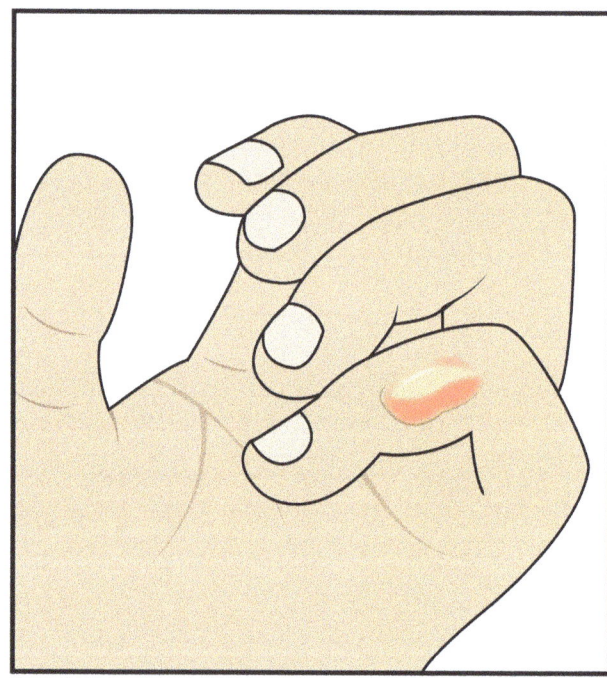

Second degree finger blister

3rd degree: deep tissue destruction, with dry, white or charred appearance, little or no pain (*Clean with soap & water, remove dead loose skin with sterile tweezers*) …
seek medical care, needs hospitalization, with IV fluids, nutritional supplements, and possible skin grafting)

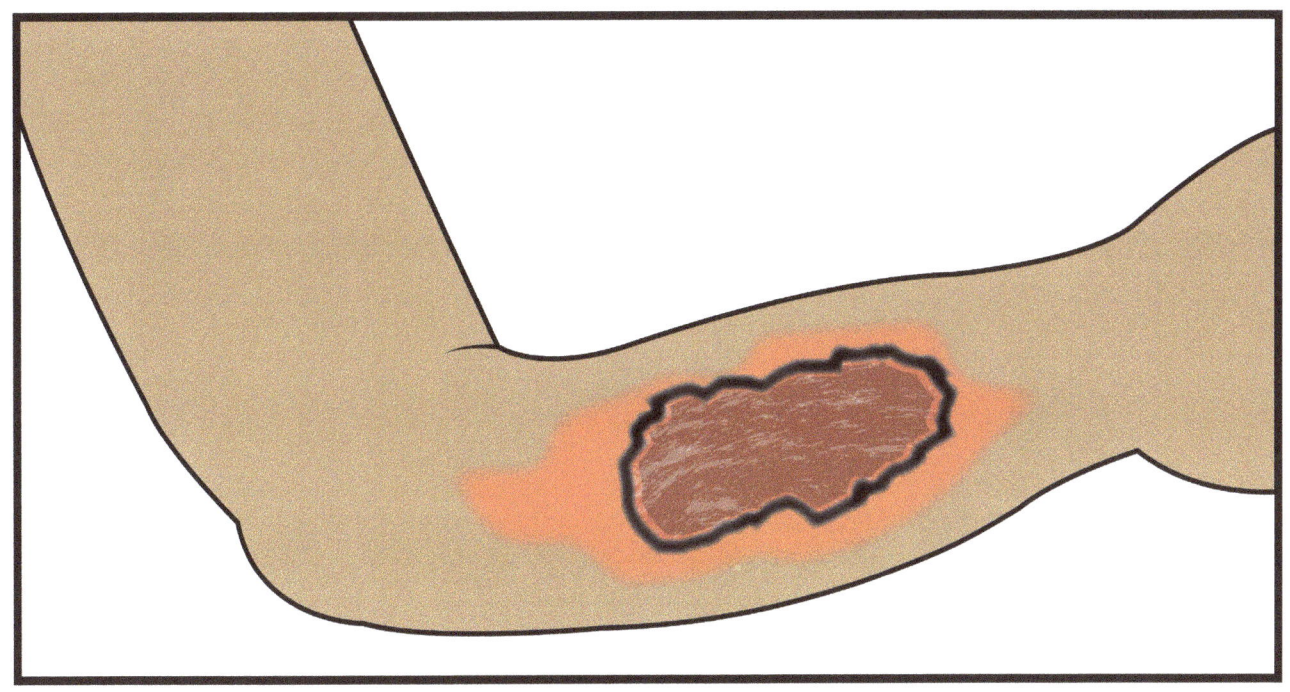

3rd degree arm burn
Electrical burn: never approach victim until sure the power is off...
Call Emergency Rescue team and electrical company immediately

C. Eye injury:
foreign body, dust, blunt trauma, plant material.

Do not rub... flush with eyewash to remove loose dirt or foreign matter, place cool wet compresses over both eyes,

*seek medical care, patch affected eye during transport.

Eye burn: (chemical): know the name of the chemical. Alkalis like ammonia and clorox are more dangerous than acids: (*Flush with cool running water for 15-30 minutes, then use eyewash drops every minute for an additional 5-10 minutes. Cover both eyes to reduce movement. *seek medical care*)

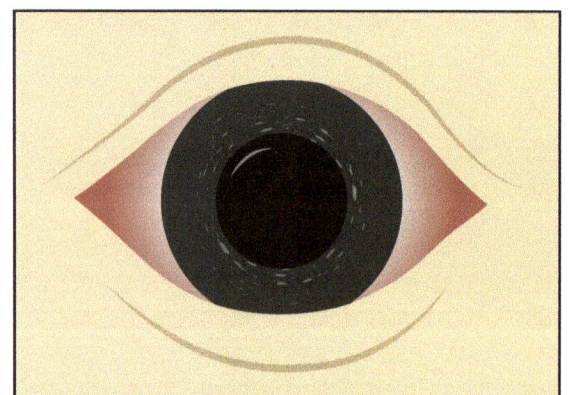

Red eye

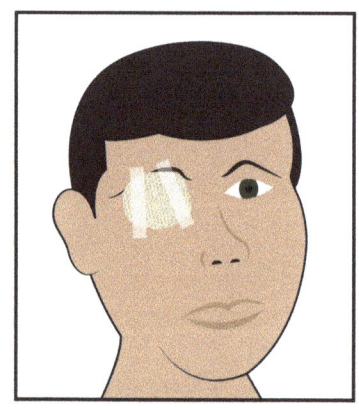

Eye patch

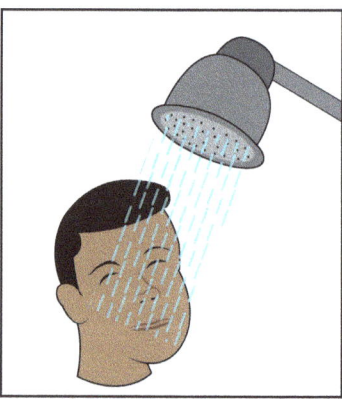

Eye wash shower

Eye penetration: entry of object into the eyeball or rupture due to blunt trauma. The pupil may be irregular & the iris may be skewed to one side.

Do not flush, patch both eyes and seek medical help immediately

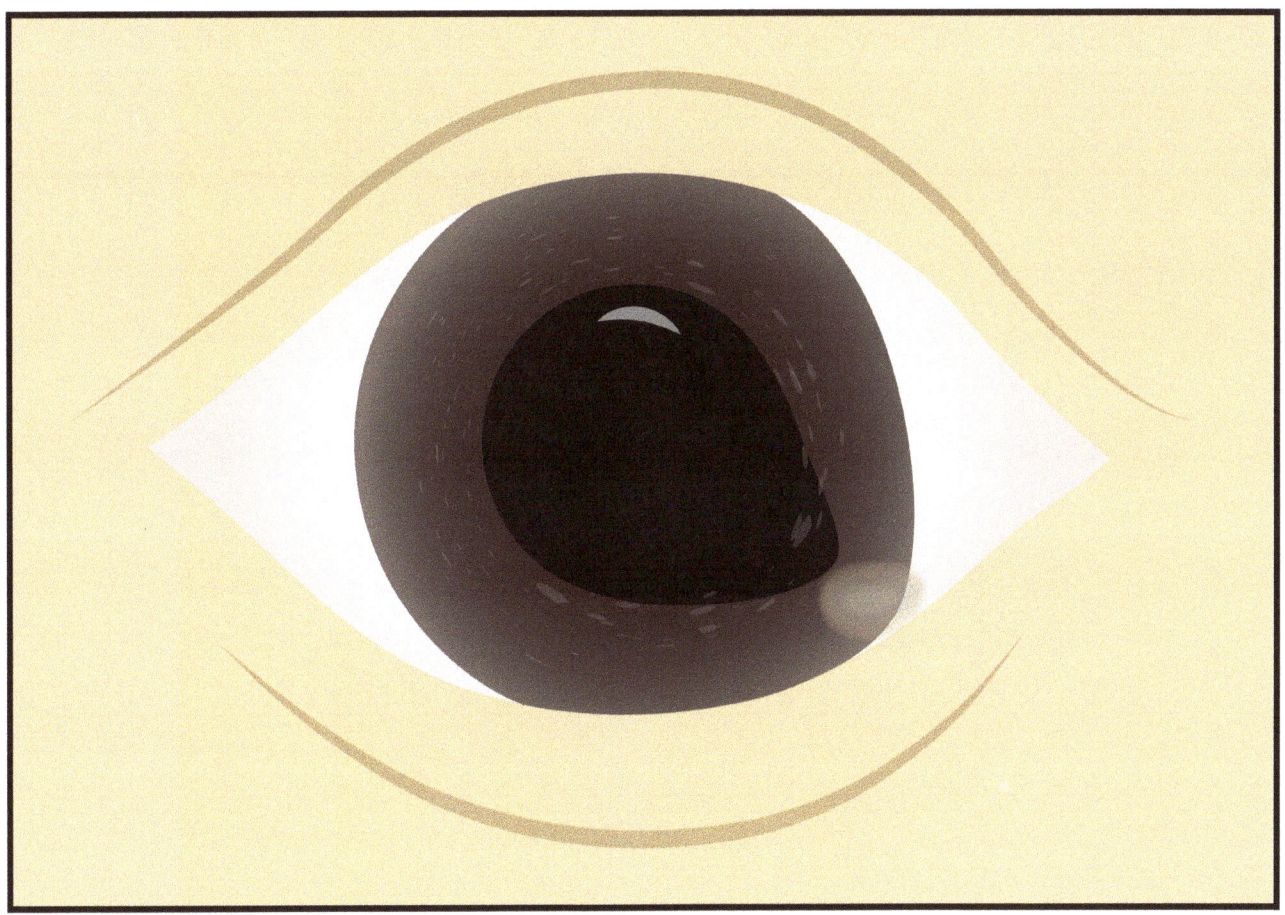

Eye penetration

D. Mouth and teeth injuries:

toothache: *chew a clove for temporary analgesia.* lip penetration, tongue puncture, lost tooth/teeth... *clear the breathing passages, insert cold sterile gauze to control bleeding, bite down for pressure, apply tincture of yarrow if needed, chew on clove for temporary analgesia; apply antibiotic ointment and new sterile dressing,*

*seek dental care

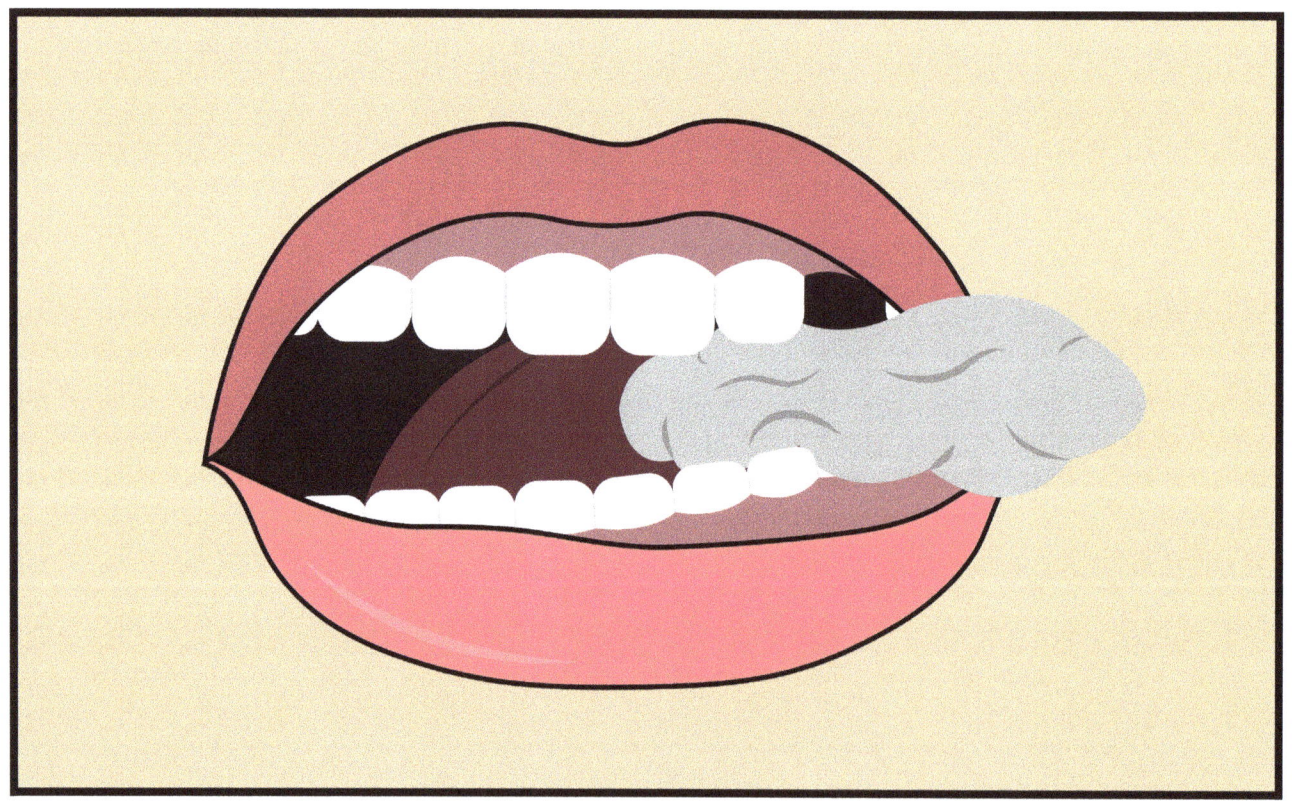

Mouth teeth injury

E. Animal bites: Assess the situation

Apply pressure to *stop bleeding, wash with soap and water, clean with antiseptic wipes and apply peroxide then antibiotic, then sterile bandage,*

*seek medical care for possible rabies or tetanus inoculation

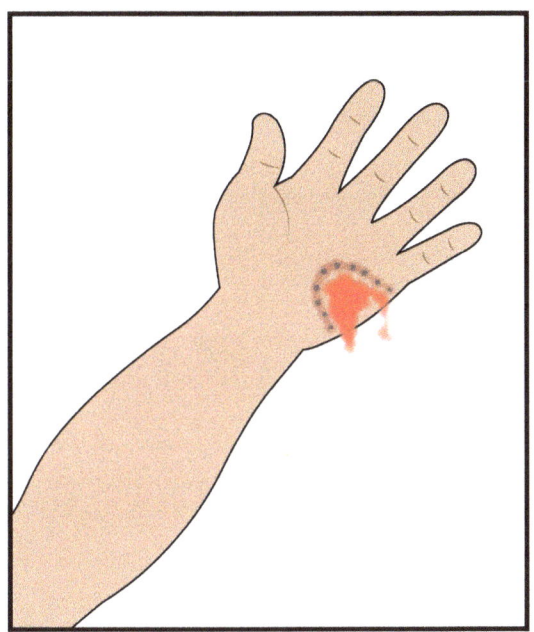

Animal bite hand

Animal bite foot

F. Perforation

2 open wounds, entry and exit(limb), entry into an organ (eye), bone exposure (scalp, limb) **seek medical care

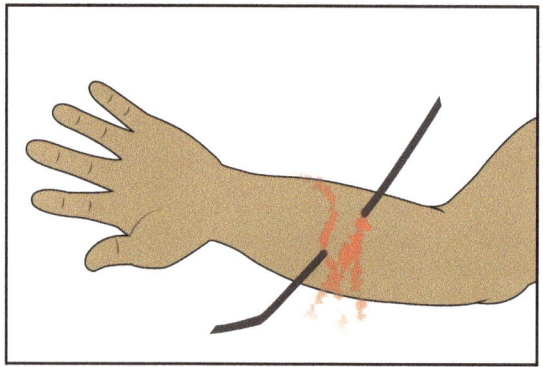

Perforating wound forearm

G. Amputation:

note body part, save it and carry it to the emergency room if possible, condition time since incident, stop bleeding with elevation, apply direct heavy pressure with cloth or heavy bandage X 15 minutes, check for shock !

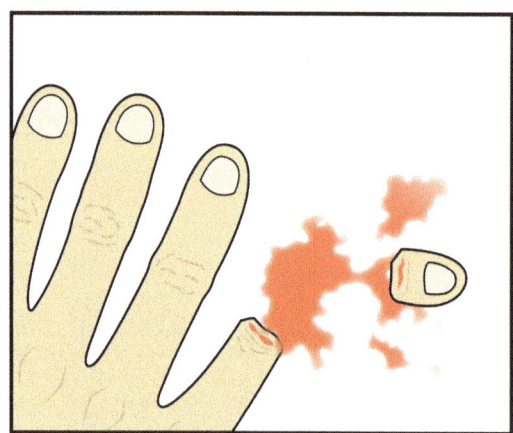

Amputated tip of little finger

** seek medical care

12. Closed wound:

<u> check for possible internal bleeding and/or organ damage</u>
1. Light-headed, dizziness, fainting, (blood loss)
2. worsening abdominal pain (liver or spleen)
3. Appearance of large area of deep purple skin (hemorrhage, hematoma, ecchymosis)
4. Swelling, tightness & pain in a limb or body part
5. Headache & loss of consciousness (brain)

A. Muscle strain:
stretch or small tear in muscle or tendon (neck, back, thigh).

(apply ice pack, arnica, elevate and rest)

B. Muscle sprain:
partial or complete tear in ligaments and tissues at the joint (ankle, knee, wrist, fingers)
(apply ice pack, elevate, seek medical care (Xray /MRI diagnostics if swelling and pain persist more than 24 hours without improvement)

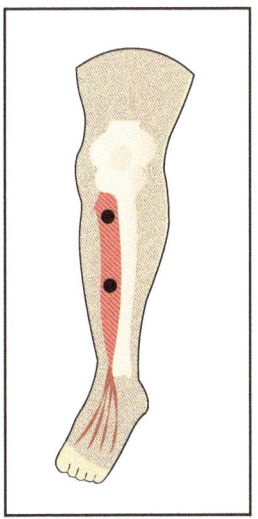

Leg muscle sprain

C. Cramp:

painful sudden contraction of muscles caused by fatigue, dehydration, and strain... (*massage, apply warm pack, elevate, hydrate*)

D. Dislocated joint:

use splint to immobilize the joint; apply ice pack; seek medical help

E. Fracture:

broken, chipped or cracked bone...(*immobilize and apply splint, do not try to realign, apply cold ice pack wrapped in cloth (not directly to skin), elevate injured area above level of the heart,* treat for shock if imminent): **seek medical care

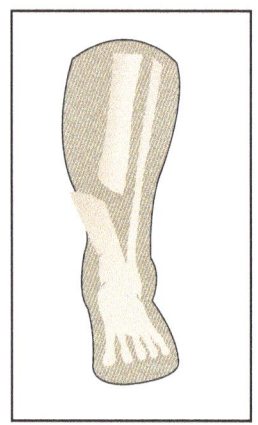
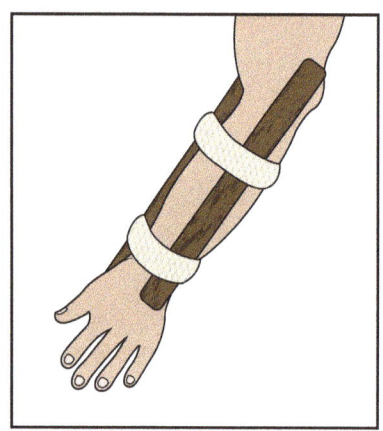
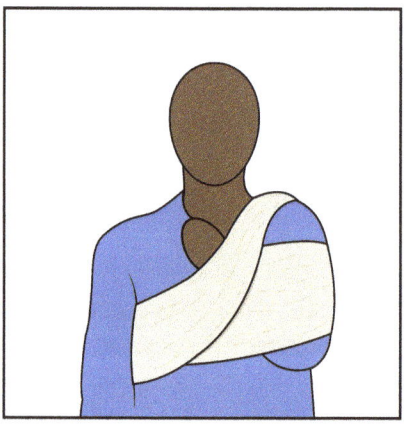

Fractured leg tibia   Forearm in splint   Left arm in sling

F. Crush injury:

impact with heavy equipment, car accident, serious fall, large animal kick, collision *(immobilize, apply wet, cold compress, if limb involved elevate to level above the heart,*

**seek medical help immediately)

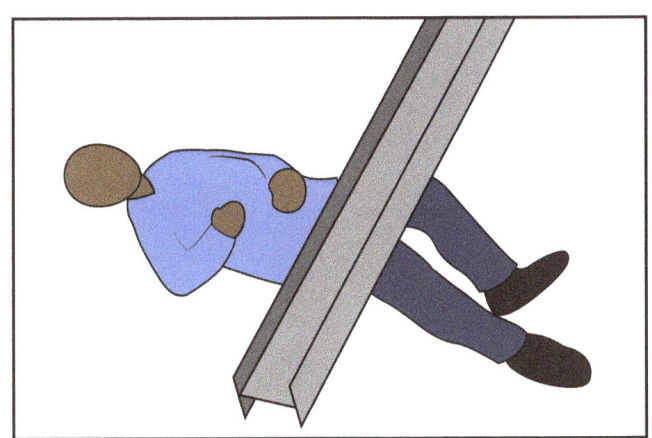

Crush injury to body / steel girder

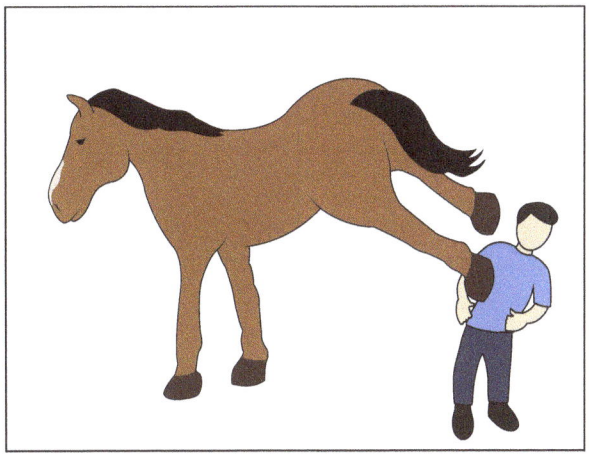

horse kick to the body

Note: Infections with fever (sepsis, blood infections, pneumonia, kidney infection, prolonged gastritis) headache, from severe injury may be unresponsive to topical or oral treatments and will require hospitalization.

** When any doubt exists seek medical care

C. Severe: (life threatening)

13. Breathing/ respiratory distress/heart attack...
check for ABC (airway, breathing, circulation)

Breathing Difficulty: Tilt the head back, lift the chin, check for breathing. <u>If not breathing</u>, pinch nose shut, place mouth over victim's mouth, give 2 gentle breaths, check to see if chest rises, then repeat 12 times, recheck breathing every 5-10 seconds; check pulse by placing fingertips along the neck groove beside the Adam's apple or on the wrist in the groove just below the base of the thumb, if pulse present but not breathing then continue rescue breathing; if no pulse and not breathing,

**call for medical help (911) and start CPR.

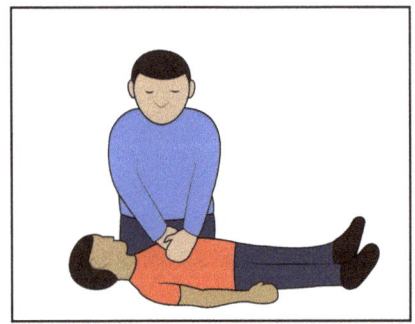 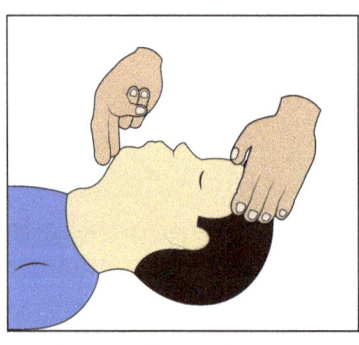 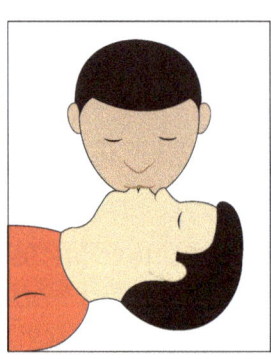

Chest compressions   Open the airway   Mouth-to-Mouth Breathing

Basic CPR: (Cardio Pulmonary Resuscitation)

<u>Infant:</u>   *Place two fingertips of one hand on the center of the chest on the breastbone; push the chest down 1 1/2 inches and let rise completely; repeat 30 times, then cover the infant's nose and mouth with your mouth and give 2 gentle breaths, watch the chest rise, repeat the sequence 3 times per minute.*

<u>Adult:</u> *Compression: place heel of one hand on the center of the victim's chest, put the other hand on top of the first with fingers interlaced, keep arms straight with shoulders*

over the hands; push the chest down 2 inches and let rise completely, then push down again 30 times, then pinch the victim's nose shut, cover mouth with your mouth and give 2 breaths (watch chest rise and fall), repeat 30 compressions then 2 breaths (full sequence 3 times per minute), until help arrives or victim revives.

AED: (Automated External Defibrillator).(requires some training). Use if victim is unresponsive, not breathing, no pulse. Power on, place electrodes right one between the nipple and collarbone, left one outside the nipple just below the armpit; press analyse button, device will tell when to deliver shock.

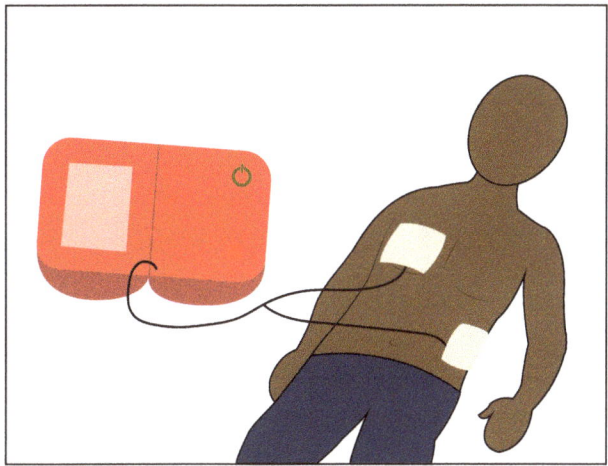

automated external defibrillator wired to the chest

14. Shock/ Anxiety attack/ Anaphylaxis (severe allergic reaction):

Due to serious injury, loss of blood, multiple stings or bites, poisoning, drug reaction or overdose,

food reaction, hazardous chemical reaction: Symptoms are sudden irritability, rapid weak pulse, rapid breathing then wheezing; ashy, cool, moist skin; excessive thirst, nausea and vomiting, drowsiness, loss of consciousness...

**Call for medical help immediately;*

Elevate legs, reassure and rest comfortably, control any external bleeding, nothing to eat or drink.

15. Choking:
if unconscious, **call for medical help.

A. Infant: place baby face down on lap with head lower than chest, hold steady with forearm, and deliver 4 rapid but light blows to back between the shoulder blades... if not working, turn baby face up on lap, place two fingers above the navel below the ribs and push into the abdomen; repeat in rapid succession... if not working, begin Rescue Breathing.

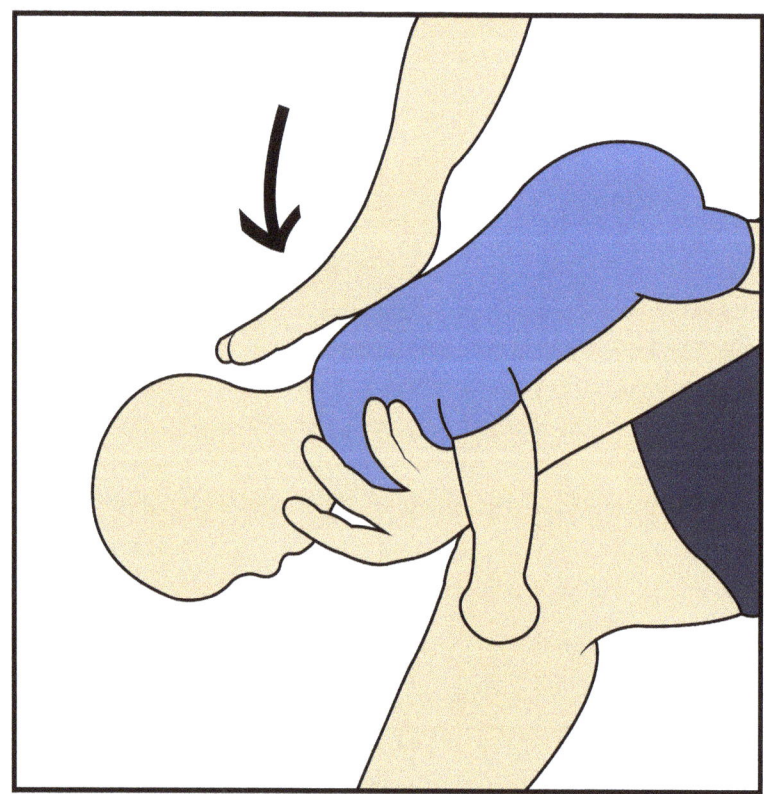

Choking infant face down over the knee

A. Choking Child or Adult:

wrap one arm around the victim's waist, make a fist, place thumb knuckle just above the navel below the breastbone, grasp your fist with the other hand, press fist into the victim's abdomen with a quick upward thrust, repeat to dislodge the object... until object is coughed up, victim starts to breathe, or if victim becomes unconscious... start CPR.

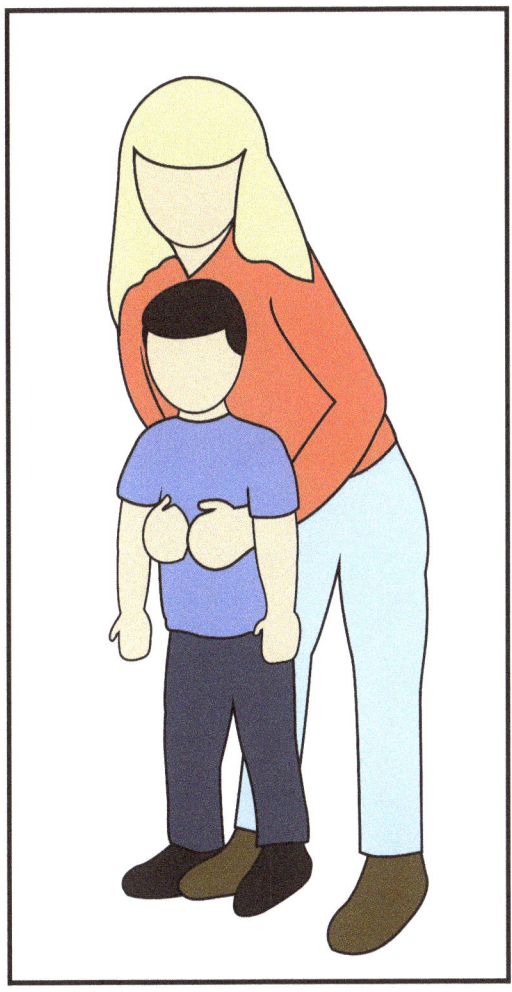

Choking child or adult

16. Poisoning:

may be swallowed, injected or absorbed through the skin; (early) see burns around lips or mouth, chemical odor breath, contracted or dilated pupils; (later) fever, nausea, vomiting, abdominal pain, diarrhea. *Drink water or milk if conscious, maintain open airway for breathing, call poison control center (1-800 222 1222) and (911) for instructions, apply CPR if necessary, transport to hospital immediately, carry the container of poison for identification...*Carbon monoxide can result from a running car engine, a wood, coal or charcoal fire, or a faulty oil burner located in a poorly-ventilated space. Lips, skin and fingernails may be pink or bright red.

(Do not induce vomiting if victim is comatose or convulsing.

(Fresh air immediately, begin CPR, seek emergency medical help.)

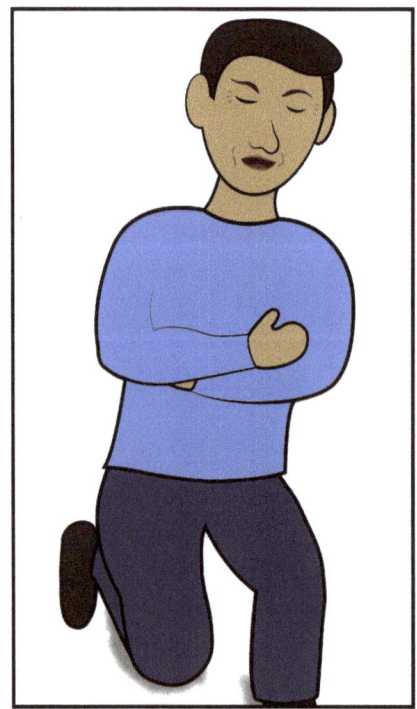

Poisoning

17. Seizure:

initial headache, agitation or blank stare, followed by rhythmic convulsions, up-rolling eyes... Do not restrain or insert anything into mouth, remove hazardous objects from the area, loosen neck clothing, turn victim onto the left side to facilitate vomiting away from the lungs, monitor pulse and breathing until seizure stops. **Call for medical help, if first seizure, if lasting more than 2-5 minutes, multiple seizures, if pregnant, head injury or diabetic. Check for ID bracelet with instructions.

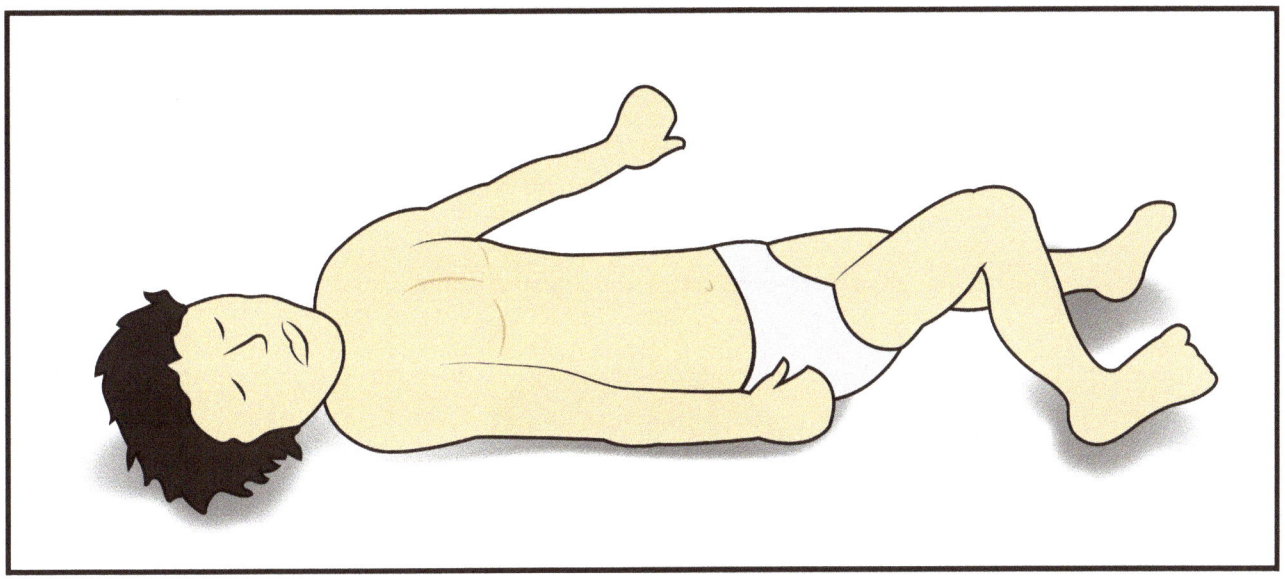

Seizure

18. Diabetic emergency:

Symptoms: Dry mouth, excessive thirst, weak, rapid pulse, fruity breath, stomach pain, vomiting, unresponsive may be high blood sugar. If known diabetic,*call personal doctor for instructions or call medical help.

Symptoms: Headache, agitation, confusion, rapid pulse, cold, clammy skin, sweating, shaking, fainting/seizure may be low blood sugar. (Give 4 ounces of orange juice, or hard candy, or 2 teaspoons sugar.

If in doubt, give sugar, low blood sugar is life-threatening, high sugar is not...

19. Stroke:

(a serious decrease in blood flow to a vital part of the brain)... weakness and numbness of one side of face, arm and/or leg, smoothing of side of forehead, droopy eyebrow, drooping corner of mouth, difficulty speaking, blurred vision, headache, dizziness, confusion, may lose consciousness or bowel and bladder control.

(Check airway if unconscious, place victim on one side to let fluid drain out of mouth, **call medical help immediately, offer comfort and assurance, monitor breathing and pulse. Nothing to eat or drink until help arrives)

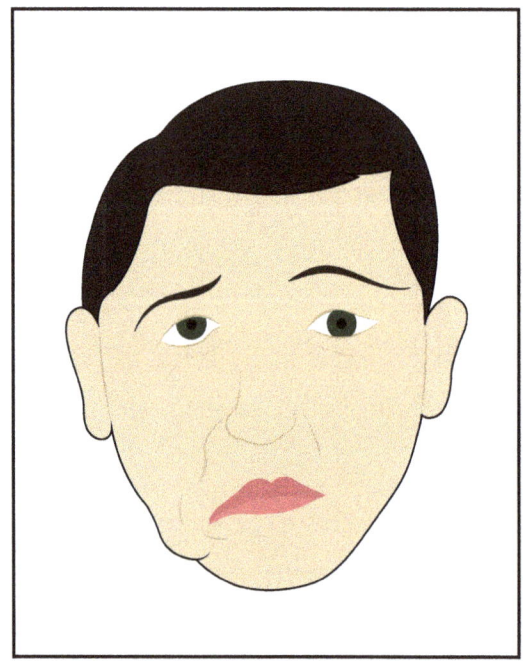

Stroke side of face sagging

20. Head, neck and spine injuries:

damage to both bone and soft tissue (brain and spinal cord), *(immobilize head neck and spine with in-line stabilization = hold head in both hands in line with body and support it until help arrives)*

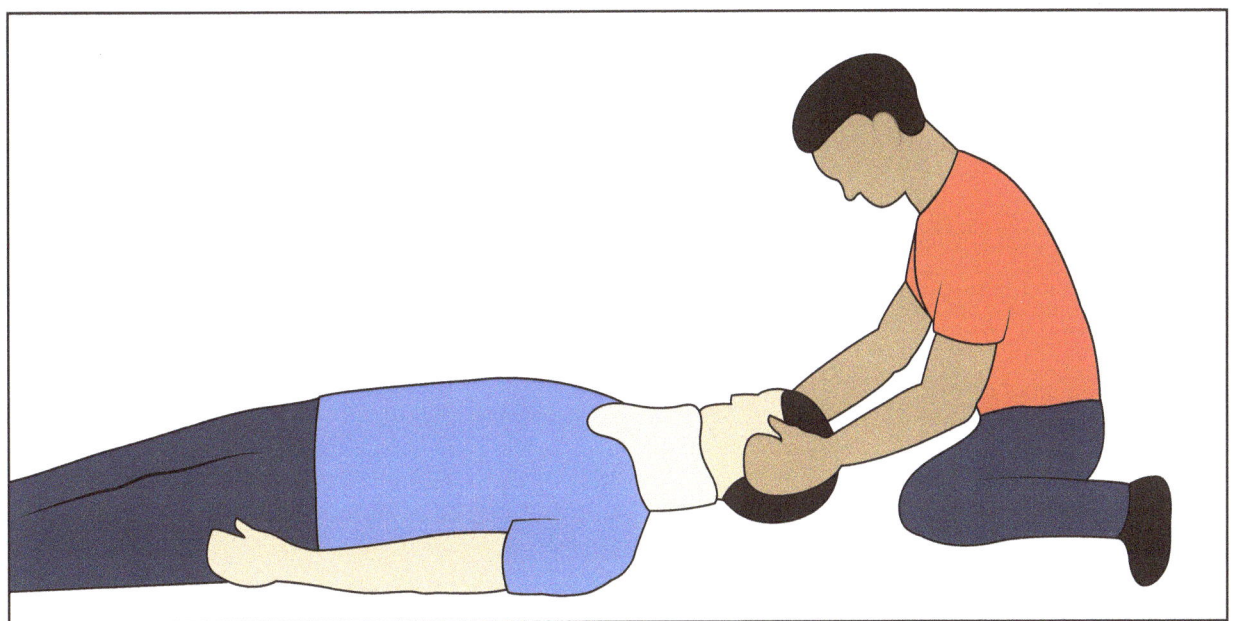

Head stabilization

www.ingramcontent.com/pod-product-compliance
Lightning Source LLC
Chambersburg PA
CBHW041131280526
45792CB00013B/2381